The Fruits of Organic Fasting

How to Rejuvenate yourself by DNA Regeneration

Nathan Gustafsson

Table of Contents

Introduction

The concept of fasting is not a new phenomenon. In ancient Greece, Pythagoras, Hippocrates, among other stalwarts of science and philosophy of those times, raved about its physical, mental, and spiritual benefits. Many of the eastern cultures, including Hinduism, Buddhism, Jainism, and others, have fasting days and periods every month to understand, appreciate, and benefit from the power of reasonable abstinence. These are followed by devout Hindus, Buddhists, and followers of Jainism even today.

Judaism exhorts its followers to fast on days such as Yom Kippur or the Day of Atonement. In Islam, the month-long Ramadan fast is observed very strictly even in the modern era. Eastern Orthodox Christian sects and Roman Catholics have a 40-day Lent period before Easter during which time they abstain from eating meats or certain types of foods. This 40-day fasting period is believed to align with the 40 days of fasting that Christ undertook in the desert. In more primitive cultures in the US such as those followed by Native Americans, fasting was a form of sacrifice to appease angry gods and deities.

Fasting was a novel kind of protest that was popularized by Mahatma Gandhi, an Indian freedom fighter who used this method very effectively to create positive social and political changes in India. His longest fasting episode lasted 21 days! Fasting might have had religious and/or political roots to achieve various ends and means. Yet, today, there are multiple research studies conducted that prove fasting is good for physical and mental health in addition to your religious health.

Dr. Herbert Sheldon is one of the pioneers of therapeutic fasting methods which gained in popularity since the 19th century. Dr. Sheldon established Dr. Shelton's Health School in 1928 in San Antonio, Texas. He is supposed to have helped over 40,000 patients to fight against diseases and become healthier than before by employing his 'water fast' method.

In the UK, Nature Cure Clinics opened all over the country which popularized fasting as a method to cure diseases and remain healthy. It is important to note that all the accepted forms of fasting were moderate in approach and included various forms of exercises, exposure to sunlight, and a positive attitude for success.

Today, there is little doubt that there are various benefits of fasting. Many of the known benefits have been substantiated by scientific research and study. This book is aimed at giving you the list of these benefits and the ways you can leverage the power of these benefits so as to improve the quality of your life. So, go ahead and learn more about the fabulous advantages of fasting and how to include organic foods so as to optimize the benefits.

Chapter One: Importance and Benefits of Fasting

The study and research on the efficiency of various fasting methods and all the benefits of fasting are still taking place and a lot more needs to be done on that front. While there is no abundance of research work done in this realm, there are ample studies which have proven the benefits of fasting on animal health and these hold promise for human health as well.

Moreover, if fasting can be done under strict medical supervision and within reasonable limits, there are hardly any contraindications except, perhaps, existing medical conditions. It is always important to consult your physician before you choose to embark on any fasting methods to leverage its benefits.

What is Fasting ?

Fasting is a process in which you choose to refrain from the intake of food, drink, or a combination of both for a specified period of time. You could choose to fast partially in which you abstain from a certain type of food (like meats) or drink only liquids and abstain from all types of solid foods. If done in the correct manner, you can reap benefits.

The human body gets into a fasting mode only 7-8 hours after the last meal. The 7-8 hours is the time taken by the body to completely utilize the nutrition from the last meal. After this period, the body draws energy from the glucose stored in muscles and liver. When this stored glucose is also finished up, then the body reaches out to the accumulated fat for energy.

However, energy from fat is used up for up to a certain extent after which proteins are broken down to release energy. When the body reaches out to proteins for energy needs, it usually means you are in a starvation mode and that is not good for you. Starvation mode happens when fasting lasts several days.

Now, let us look at the benefits of fasting.

Fasting and Curing of Diseases

While fasting may not directly help in curing diseases, it helps the body to focus on self-healing. The following things are responsible for the self-healing process:

- The body's vital organs are completely and thoroughly rested

- Fasting prevents further intake of foods which get digested in the intestines and 'poisons' the sick body even further

- Fasting facilitates the complete removal of putrefying bacteria and other digestive organisms from the digestive tract

- The organs involved in eliminating undigested solids and liquids are given time and energy to catch up with their overload of work and truly eliminate all the toxins from the body

- Fasting helps the body get back some kind of normalcy in its biochemical and physiological balances and secretions.

- Fasting facilitates the breaking down of 'diseased' cells and tissues, effusions, deposits, exudates, and all other kinds of abnormal growths and extensions.

- The youthful state of cells, tissues, and organs is restored and rejuvenated during the period of fasting

- Energy is conserved, as a lot of needless wasting of energy connected with food-related physiological and biochemical functions is done away with. This conserved energy is channeled in a more productive way toward cell repair and restoration leading to enhanced self-healing

- Fasting increases the power of digestion and assimilation

- The overall functioning of the body is increased

As fasting is a form of rest, a housecleaning kind of process takes place for all of the body's biochemical and physiological functions. Therefore, fasting can be an efficient treatment process for all kinds of diseases. It is, of course, very important to remember to use therapeutic fasting only under medical supervision.

In addition to helping in treating diseases in the above ways, there are multiple studies which prove the efficacy of fasting in the treatment of the following diseases and healing some of the body systems:

Cancer – Fasting is believed to be helpful in enhancing the effectiveness of chemotherapy. Multiple studies have since revealed the changes in the glucose levels due to fasting helps in improving the efficacy of chemotherapy treatments against tumors. When there is no calorie consumption for a limited and defined period of time, plenty of changes take place in the protective nature of body cells and this is very useful during chemotherapy.

Fasting is also believed to reduce the toxicity associated with chemotherapy while sensitizing the 'cancer' cells to the chemicals that are being infused into the body. This sensitization is proven to encourage the breakdown and deterioration of these cancer cells. Again, it would be very important to point out here that this kind of therapeutic fasting has to take place only under strict medical supervision and only on the advice and recommendation of qualified medical professionals.

While fasting, the human body is proven to produce less IGF-1, growth factor 1 which works similar to insulin. This compound is believed to facilitate the spread of cancer cells throughout the body. Reduced production of IGF-1 while fasting, therefore, helps in reducing the risk of growth and spread of cancer cells. Fasting, therefore, not only cleanses your body of tumor cells, but also eliminates the hormone believed to be responsible for their proliferation.

Cardiovascular Diseases – Intermittent fasting or fasting for short periods of time, which is possible through reduced meal frequencies is known to facilitate the production of brain-derived neurotrophic factor (BDNF), a compound that is responsible for regulating cardiovascular health. Multiple studies in the area of BDNF and fasting have been conducted and many of them have shown a direct positive connection to the upkeep of the health of your heart, your blood pressure, body mass, insulin sensitivity, and triglyceride levels.

Levels of triglycerides in the blood reduce during fasting. This fatty cholesterol in the blood has the potential to increase the risk of narrowed arteries, putting your cardiovascular health at risk. Fasting helps in reducing this risk. In some animal health studies, it was proved that the performance of heart muscles increased significantly, free radicals were decreased, and growth of blood vessels inside the heart got better with intermittent fasting. This study holds much promise for the health of the human heart as well.

Improved Insulin Sensitivity – When you fast, you are restricted intake of sugar into your body which reduces the production of insulin. When the production of insulin decreases, people with insulin resistance become more sensitive to it. Moreover, increased fat accumulation is also believed to cause insulin resistance. Fasting reduces fat accumulation, thereby facilitating improved insulin sensitivity.

In the initial days of any fasting regimen, the sugar level drops significantly, which is a huge perk for people with hyperglycemia. While this big drop might make you feel a little tired and low on energy, the blood sugar level usually stabilizes as the fasting continues provided all other vitals remain strong and within healthy limits.

Immune System and Healing – When food is absent in the stomach, the body is able to focus on other physiological functions including repair and rejuvenation of cells and tissues, resulting in improved healing of your body and a better-performing immune system. There are research studies that have proven an improved immune system when patients have undergone therapeutic fasting under medical supervision.

The recycling and synthesis of cellular components which is a mechanism referred to as autophagy gets a boost during fasting leading to increased production of healthy cells and tissues resulting in an improved immune system, overall.

Decreased Inflammation – While inflammation can be caused by a variety of causes, an unhealthy diet is, undoubtedly, a consistent cause. Unhealthy and/or unhygienic foods can be an aggravating source for increased production of free radicals. Foods that increase the risk of inflammation include refined carbs, refined sugars, meat, alcohol, dairy charred or fried foods, etc. In addition to unhealthy diet, another major cause for the increased production of free radicals is metabolic reactions which generate free radicals like hydrogen peroxide and super-oxides.

Fasting, therefore (or giving up a few meals), can reduce inflammation caused by foods and metabolic reactions even before they start production. Moreover, fasting facilitates hormonal balance resulting in reduced inflammation as well. Multiple studies have also proven that inflammation is reduced through lowering of insulin levels and better insulin sensitivity as both these activities decrease oxidative stress.

Facilitates Anti-aging- Free radicals and increased inflammation are two big contributors to premature aging. When you fast, your body is benefited through improved hormone signaling, improved blood composition, healthy gene signaling, and less oxidative stress than before. All these factors help in reducing oxidative stress considerably, which, in turn, keeps your cells, tissues, organs, and your genes healthy even as you grow older.

Moreover, as the human body ages, foreign and human rogue cells can spread throughout the body damaging tissues and contributing to progressive diseases too. When you fast, the autophagy mechanism is promoted resulting in cell recycling through self-digestion of bad cells and regeneration of new cells.

Fasting, therefore, not only helps you digest fat but also helps you digest and get rid of malfunctioning and damaged cells, resulting in healthy cells, tissues, organs, and overall body. Fasting helps in destroying malfunctioning cells through the process of selective protection. Fasting promotes the selective protection of healthy cells and tissues and destroys unhealthy cells and tissues, thereby optimizing the physiological functioning of the human body.

Purifies the Skin and the Hair – Additionally, fasting is believed to improve the condition of your skin. How does this happen? When you eat, there is a lot of change in your blood sugar levels, which alters the collagen structure in your skin. The collagen loses strength and becomes weak, resulting in sagging skin. When you fast, the blood sugar levels are more or less kept constant which, in turn, keeps the collagen in your skin healthy, strong, and tight leaving it looking youthful even in old age.

Furthermore, fasting affect directly the quality and the vitality of the hair. As every part of the body, the hair are a living organism. Each strand of hair start with a root, called the hair root plexus. The function of this plexus is to connect the hair to the brain, mainly by sending and receiving nerve impulses. These electric signals determine the quality of the hair, by bringing more life to the root.

By gaining vitality with new fresh cells, the hair can rejuvenate itself. Each strand can breathe fluently again, so being softer and better looking from outside.

Hair loss or white hair symptoms are due to a receptor nerves failure, meaning that the connection is no strong enough to bring life to the hair root plexus. Causing depigmentation or even death of the strand.

Fasting reinforce the immune system and so the hair root plexus. Then hair can regain color, softness and strong roots.

Helps in the Prevention of Brain Damage – Due to increased life expectancy all over the world, studies on the brain and the functioning of the brain have gone up considerably. People are keen on aging gracefully keeping their physical and mental faculties working well right up to the end of their lives. Fasting appears to help promote physical and mental health in old age by preventing brain damage.

There are multiple products of metabolism and proteins that cause inflammation, especially in the brain, resulting in reduced faculties and, even severe damage. Calorie inhibition and fasting are known to restrict the production of free radicals and other harmful proteins can cause inflammatory reactions in the brain.

There is a lot of evidence which reveals that these free radicals and harmful proteins could be responsible for premature aging of the brain. The process of fasting, which helps in the reduced production of these free radicals, can help in preventing this catastrophe. In fact, fasting is believed to not only reduce the production of inflammatory and harmful cytokine but also increases the production and release of productive cytokine resulting in improved brain health even as you age leaving you in full control of your physical and mental faculties. 10

Fasting helps in faster recovery from injury – It is a natural thing to think that recovery from injury needs more glucose to the brain and the body. However, intermittent fasting in animal studies has proven that it helps in improving brain function and cell regeneration.

Fasting and Sports

Here is how intermittent fasting is believed to help athletes perform better than otherwise:

Full-day-fasts – Full day fasts consist of going completely off food and calories for 24 hours. That means, if you have had dinner on Saturday at 8 PM, then your next meal should be only at 8 PM, on Sunday. During these hours when your body is free from having to focus on digestion, it will channelize the conserved energy towards:

- Increasing levels of growth hormone
- Detoxifying the liver
- Reduced inflammation

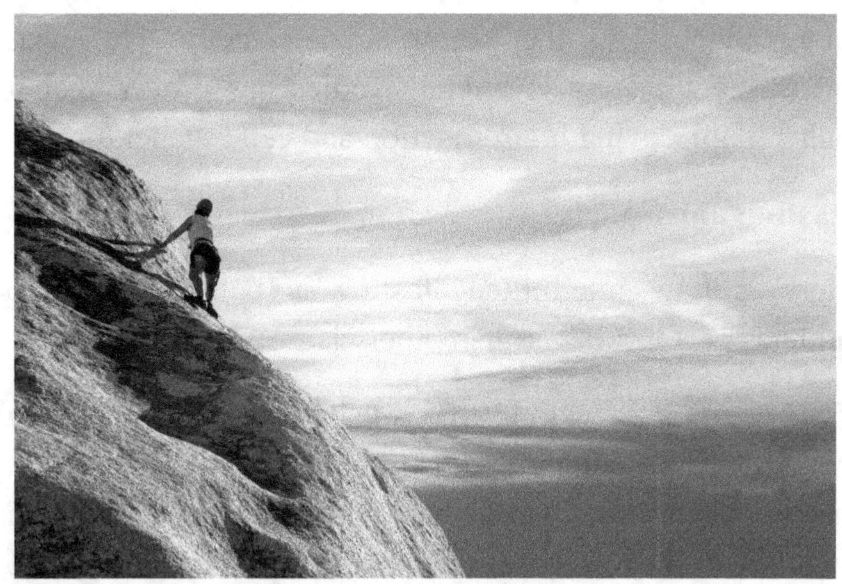

These activities help athletes in the following ways:

- Recover from small injuries received during the week
- Recover from stiff joints and other aches
- Helps athletes in weight class sports to maintain and manage their weight and body fat

However, athletes must remember to completely relax on their full fasting days. There should be minimal physical activity restricted to walking along with naps and plenty of sleep. Keeping yourself busy is a great way to keep your mind off food too.

Daily fasts – This kind involves fasting every day for 16 hours with an 8-hour window for eating. Daily fast regimens help keep your mind sharp and focused, which could be channeled to improve performance and speed of workouts and training. It is always better to skip breakfast so that you can eat dinner and being satiated before sleeping will result in improved rest. Moreover, it is always better to sleep off maximum part of the fasting period. Of course, if you need to do training during the fasting period, then you must supplement your energy sources with some form of protein supplement, perhaps, BCAA (branched chain amino acids).

Moreover, if you have a game or match during the fasting period, then it needs to be handled differently. It is recommended that all kinds of fasting with preconditions, including medical and sports-related, have to be done under strict medical supervision.

You must experience different way of fasting to really know what your body is capable, each human being is unique and will respond differently. The best way is to try and to feel the benefits and the limits of fasting on your body.

Be your own judge and be responsible for yourself.

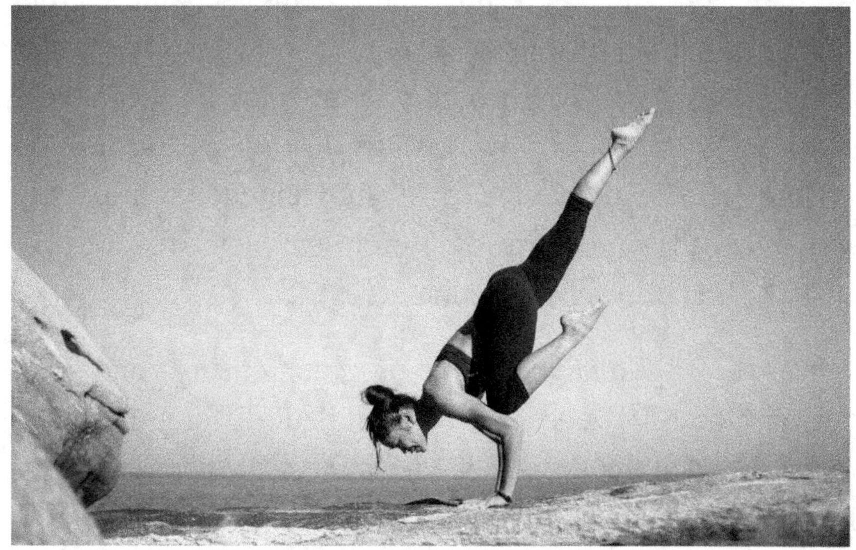

Go slowly first, step by step, and learn by experience.

Chapter Two: Importance and Benefits of Fasting Continued

Fasting and Weight Loss

Many of us would love to shed fat and remain fit and healthy. Well, there are multiple scientific studies that prove fasting can help with weight loss and weight management too. The primary reason why fasting helps you to lose weight is that you end up with a lower calorie intake. During periods of fasting, your calorie intake is almost negligible. Therefore, unless you make up for this calorie loss during times of eating, fasting is bound to help you consume fewer calories thereby helping you manage your weight.

In fact, intermittent fasting has proven to help people lose belly fat. Therefore, intermittent fasting is a great way to lose weight and fat without restricting yourself to eating less. Moreover, there are studies that reveal that intermittent fast facilitates the retention of muscle mass while using up fat for energy needs.

Therefore, intermittent fasting not only helps you lose weight by using up fat, it also helps in retaining crucial muscle mass which is essential for fitness. Another reason why intermittent fasting helps in weight loss is it makes healthy eating easy to do.

For example, the daily intermittent fasting regimen consists of eating in the 8-hour window while fasting in the 16-hour window. This means you will have to eat only 2 meals which are easier to prepare and get ready than 3 or more meals a day. The easier a diet is to follow, the higher the chances of success. Here are some important points to remember if you wish to lose weight with intermittent fasting:

Quality of food – Even if you are fasting for 16 hours, ensure you stick of whole grain, single-ingredient, and fiber-rich foods when you eat.

Calories – Keep count of your calories. It is important to eat your usual amount during the eating periods so as to keep the overall daily calorie intake at a lower level than if you were not on intermittent fasting. If you end up doubling your calorie intake during the eating periods, your calorie restriction is hardly met. So, you have to still count calories when you are following intermittent fasting regimens

Consistent efforts – Like any other diet programs, consistent and long-term efforts are required for effective results.

Patience – You have to be patient with yourself and give your body time to get adjusted to the new diet protocol.

For this, you must be consistent with your meal schedules so your body adapts easily to the fasting regimen.

Therefore, with intermittent fasting, you must still follow healthy and consistent diets and maintain a calorie deficit to achieve weight loss.

Fasting and the Nervous System

There are multiple studies which have proven beneficial effects of fasting on the workings of our nervous system. Studies conducted fasting people revealed slowing of the alpha wave and increased movement of theta waves. A situation wherein there are decreased alpha waves and increased theta waves is reflective of calm nerves and relaxed and introspective state of mind. This situation is aligned less with the normal waking state associated usually with superficial and transient thought patterns.

Similar brain wave patterns were noticed in people who were involved with Zen meditation. Therefore, such studies concluded that fasting and meditation have similar psycho-physiological effects on the brain waves resulting in calming the nerves and allowing you to reach deeper than normal waking states.

A slowing down effect on the brain functioning also reflects the slowing down of the central nervous system. This means that at the nervous system's cellular level, more complex reactions and changes must be taking place resulting in calmed nerves. An overactive nervous system is continually relaying abnormal psychic and mental stresses into our body's systems and organs, resulting in over-activity of these systems which could be the cause of disease and disorder states.

Fasting and meditative techniques are believed to remove these stress signals being continually sent to the entire body. This slowing down of stress signals allow the other organ systems of the body, such as the respiratory system, the cardiovascular system, the gastrointestinal system, etc. to revert to normal functioning.

Emotional Benefits of Fasting

An important benefit of fasting is the positive effect it has on our emotional status. During fasting, you are likely to feel highly emotional, a state which could extend into after the fasting break too. However, this heightened sense of emotion is usually positive as the fasting process cleanses your emotions.

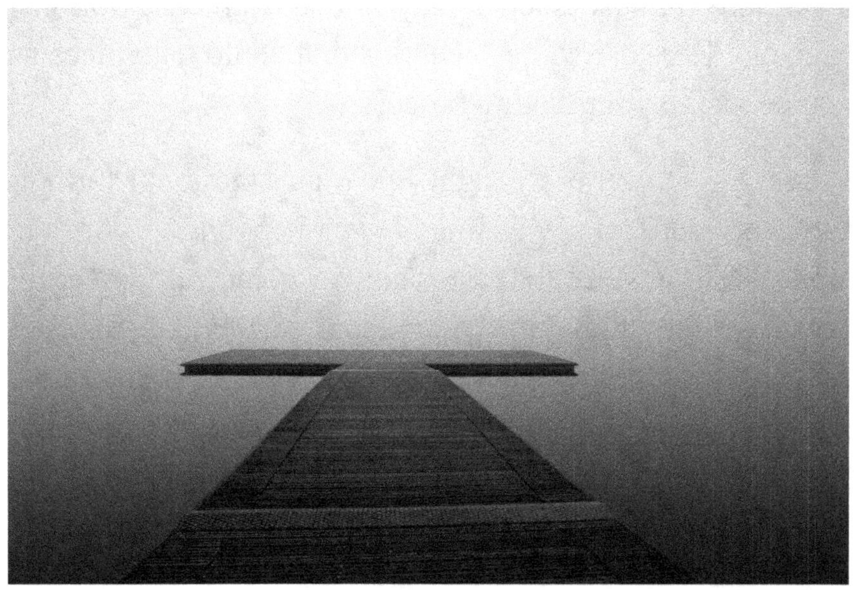

The emotional cleanse that is bound to take place during fasting is the most important reason for you to take things slowly during the fasting period. This period should ideally become a period of self-discovery. If you stick to your usual rushed schedule during the fasting periods, you are likely to miss out on this self-discovery process. You are likely to miss out an opportunity to gain a new insight or to view a nagging problem a little differently, giving you the power to find solutions that were hitherto obscure.

If you rush through your fasting period, you might miss out on the opportunity to release heavy emotional baggage that has now become so deeply embedded that you don't even realize you are carrying it. When you fast, these kinds of revelations can be had and you can potentially release such heavy and unwanted emotional baggage. Here are some scenarios that could take place as you persist in your fasting process.

Scene 1 – If you are caught up in an emotional turmoil and are wondering why this always happens to you, the most likely answer that is bound to come up is, "Well, because I am that kind of person who reacts to such situations in such a way." However, during a period of fast while you focus on your emotions instead of rushing through your life, a moment of revelation, consciously or unconsciously, might come up wherein you see your emotional turmoil in a different light.

You could see the actual reason for this turmoil without being clouded by subjectivity. You could realize that there was some old fear, an old and forgotten obstacle, or something that was preventing you from opening up. A clear answer can emerge if you allow yourself to slow down and give in to your emotions during fasting.

If you are aware of the release of tension in a conscious manner, you could take the learning and use it in other aspects of your life. Else, you can at least feel the stress lift from that aspect of your life.

Scene 2 – There could be a time when you are upset about something in your life. It could be anything ranging from being fat to having a horrible spouse to not earning enough money and so forth. While fasting, the same emotionally upsetting attitude can feel very different. You are quite likely to feel lighter about the upsetting emotion and there is usually a sense of airiness about your attitude.

You could become aware of the fact that these awful feelings are so transient that they disappear if you don't give them much thought. You could feel a sense of understanding creeping in about all the wrong things you have been doing to yourself which is resulting in these upsetting emotions. You could suddenly have an insight like, "No wonder I was feeling so awful. Look at what is around me!" These flashes can trigger remedial action from your end to improve the quality of life.

Scene 3 – You open your desk drawer and suddenly are appalled at the mess in it. You ask yourself how you managed to make such a mess in your drawer. You quickly clear it up and when you see a clean drawer at the end of the exercise, you will feel lighter, happier, and more satisfied with yourself than before. You will feel a sense of achievement.

You see, when your mind does not have to worry about the next meal and what you will be eating, then it will be freer to look at the more important things in your life and give itself time to perceive things differently. This creates clarity of thought in your mind leaving you less burdened than before. Fasting releases tension and stress leaving your body and mind to be free to do things that are as important as food.

Mental Benefits of Fasting

Fasting improves mental clarity and gets you to focus better so that you are able to work more freely, with more energy, and with more flexibility than before. With a clear thought process, you will find the ability to prioritize your work better making sure you do the most important thing first and leaving the least important ones for the last.

In fact, as you get involved deeply in your fasting regimen, you will find yourself choosing to fast before a crucial deadline so that you can focus better and do your work in an improved way. Painters and other artists are known to forego food during their creative peaks so that their mind remains focused and sharp.

Many times, it is quite difficult to draw a clear separating line between our emotional and mental states. More often than not, the emotional aspect of our life overlaps the mental aspect of our life. It is very difficult to discern between the sources of pain. For example, am I feeling sad because I had this thought or did I have this thought because I am feeling sad?

Once the source of agony is identified, it is so easy to see that all feelings were unnecessarily blown out of proportions. Fasting helps you see this source and also helps you lead a more fulfilled, happier, and a more aware life than before.

Spiritual Benefits of Fasting

This is one of the most fabulous effects of fasting. Fasting has a powerful influence on your spiritual journey. When you fast, you feel the power to look inward and focus on what is happening within you rather than outside of you. Fasting slows down all our processes and you become quiet and silent. The silent quality time you spend with yourself opens up inner aspects that were hitherto considered non-existent. You will find it easy to connect with your inner being.

With little or no residue of heavy foods inside your system, the potential energy in your body and mind is channeled towards the inner self and you feel lighter than before. This sense of lightness helps you realize the ordinariness and limitations of the physical realities around you along with the worldly things they hold. You begin to realize the power of things beyond human senses and comprehension.

Your ability to pray and meditate gets better and clearer than before. Your prayers will be based less on worldly things and more about the other-worldly requirements. You will find it easier to achieve higher states of consciousness when you choose to abstain from eating and drinking. You will find it easier and more open to receiving messages from beings who occupy higher planes of consciousness than before. You will be able to feel their love for you.

You will know intuitively that you are loved and supported right through your life. This knowledge will empower you to believe more in the presence of the divine which, in turn, will help you release your stresses. You will realize that there is someone higher up and more capable than you who is looking down at you with compassion and love.

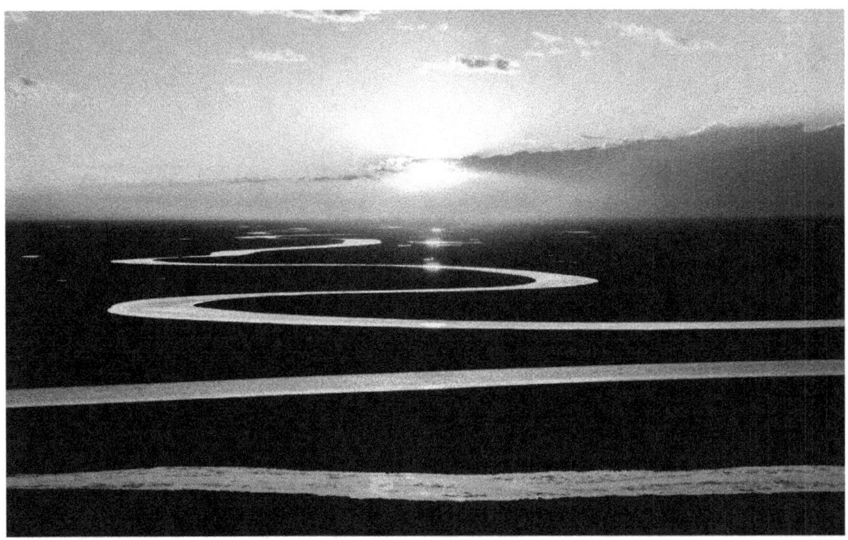

You will be able to see the higher purpose of this life and this will give you the strength to go through the struggles of human life with dignity without feeling cowed down and weakened. Every one of your experiences will become personal and unique including the routine ones that you do day in and day out. You will become more mindful of all the things happening in your life and you will notice even the most subtle elements that are creating joy and happiness for you. You will fill your life with gratitude.

Fasting is a wonderful way to live a happier, healthier, and spiritually fulfilled life. Food is an essentiality, no doubt. However, we need to let our body and mind become free from the rigors of basic living needs so that they can use the conserved and accrued energy to reach higher levels of life.

Chapter Three: Importance and Benefits of Organic Foods

Now that you know the amazing benefits of fasting, let us look at organic foods and their benefits in this chapter. In the next chapter, we can look at combining the two so that you are doubly benefited through organic fasting.

What are Organic Foods?

Organic foods are produced without the use of man-made fertilizers and chemicals. Organic produce is grown and/or reared without the use of pesticides, food additives, and growth regulators. Organic foods also exclude genetically modified organisms (GMOs) and by-products of GMOs.

Organic farming is focused on nature. This means no use of artificial chemicals and fertilizers which can pollute the soil and the water under the soil, which could percolate to all the water resources underground. Organic farming includes increased use of wildlife produce and increased biodiversity.

Benefits of Organic Produce

Generally, consumers, manufacturers, and farmers of organic produce say that organic produce is more beneficial to humanity than that produced with chemicals and genetic modifications. Here are some of the benefits listed below:

Antioxidant Capacity – Multiple studies have been conducted on the effects and influences of antioxidants from various types of foods on the physiological and biochemical functions of the human body. Most of these studies have revealed that the anti-oxidative capabilities of organic foods are much better than non-organic foods.

Scientists opine that this result could be because of the fact that in organic foods, there are no chemicals and foreign additives that negatively impact the working of vitamins, minerals, and other elements present in fruits and vegetables. These 'pure' nutrients are better equipped to fight and prevent diseases such as premature aging, heart diseases, cancer, cognitive diseases, vision problems, etc.

Therefore, the nutrients from organic foods are more empowered with anti-oxidative properties than the nutrients in non-organic foods resulting in improved health in general.

Reduced Effects of Pesticides – One of the most important benefits of choosing organic foods over non-organic foods is the fact there are no pesticides used in the former. Artificially manufactured pesticides seem like a necessary element to keep out pests and bugs from destroying and harming crops. However, these pesticides are made with very harmful chemicals, most of which can cause damage to human beings.

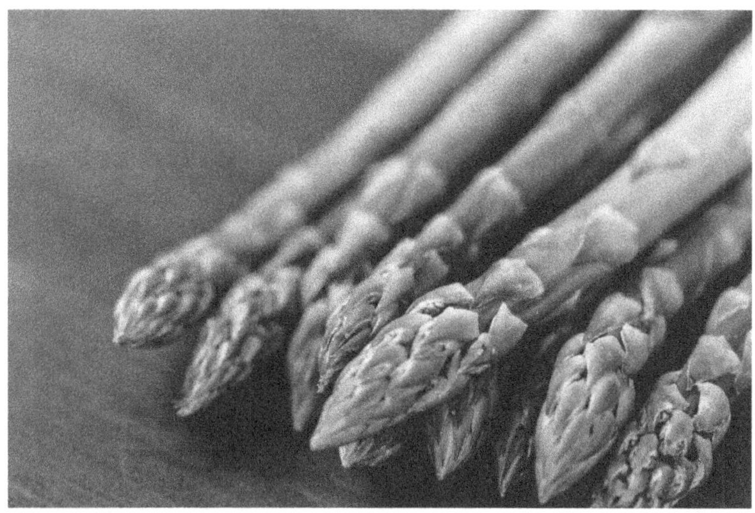

A common compound found in most pesticides is organophosphorus, a chemical and artificial compound that is absolutely not needed by the human body. Yet, nearly 80% of this compound found in our bodies is from consuming foods produced and grown with pesticides.

Organophosphorus is not just a non-essential compound for humans but is also connected to multiple developmental disorders such as ADHD and autism. It is no wonder that there are many people who choose to go organic in an attempt to let their kids grow in a healthy way without the toxins from pesticides affecting them negatively. Using pesticides for growing traditional food is a great reason for you to switch to organic.

Improved Heart Health – The more grass cattle graze, the more is the incidence of conjugated linoleic acid (CLA), a product that is found in animal meats and products. CLA is a fatty acid is very good for the health of your heart and enhances cardiovascular protection. It is found in higher concentrations in breast milk and in the meats and meat products of animals that have been reared in a free and non-caged environment.

Improved Immunity – In recent decades, driven by increased poverty across the globe, farmers, manufacturers, and scientists have been on a roll with regards to genetic modification. Yes, being able to grow six times larger tomatoes and potatoes than the naturally found ones can, perhaps, solve some of the hunger problems of the world temporarily.

However, the studies on the effects of genetic modification are still in the nascent stage. The long-term effects of consuming genetically modified foods are still unclear. However, animals have been tested with genetically modified foods and some scary results have been revealed including:

- Lowered immunity
- Increased birth mortality
- Sexual dysfunction
- Cancers
- Increased sensitivity to allergens

Most advocates of organic produce request you to be cautious about consuming genetically modified foods as the long-term effects on human health are not yet very clear.

Increased Resistance to Antibiotics – As more and more people are becoming sensitive to their health, there is an increased incidence of taking sufficient precautions in the form of vaccines and antibiotics for protection against new strains of bacteria. The thing about non-organic food produce, especially meats obtained from animals reared in feed houses and traditional farms, is that antibiotics are regularly given to these animals and plants to prevent the spread of infections and diseases.

So, when you eat produce from such places, you are, in effect, consuming extra antibiotics which could result in increased resistance. This overdosing of antibiotics through the food you consume is bound to result in a weak immune system and repeated such happenings can potentially reshape your system so much so that it may not be able to protect you at all. It must be remembered that growers of organic produce are prohibited from using antibiotics in any of their processes.

Improved Overall Health – Organic foods are grown and prepared without the use of chemical and/or artificial fertilizers. Therefore, these kinds of foods do not contain even traces of any harmful chemicals that can damage human cells and tissues. Organic food growers use only natural fertilizers like manure to enrich the soil and keep out pests. These kinds of natural manures may be a bit smelly, but are a much safer option than man-made chemical pesticides and fertilizers. When you consume foods grown with natural manures, you are bound to be unaffected by any harmful chemicals resulting in overall good health.

Improved Taste – This could be a subjective point of discussion. Some people believe that organic produce tastes better than traditionally grown produce as the process used is all natural with no additives or chemicals included in the process. Moreover, organic produce is usually sold locally, which means you truly get fresh produce straight from the farm or feed house without it having to travel any carbon miles.

There will not be any need for refrigeration until you take the produce home and need to keep it for a day or two. Organic foods may not have seen a refrigerator before the one in your home.

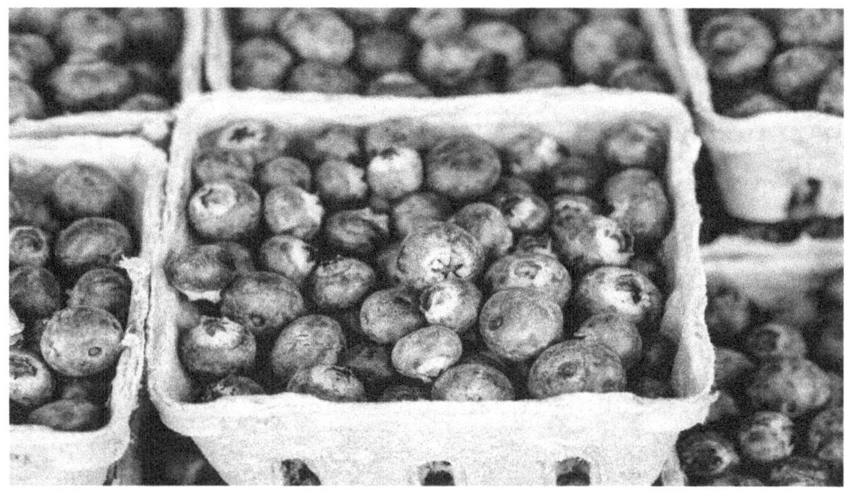

On the other hand, traditionally grown foods are invariably frozen, packed (with preservatives, perhaps), shipped, and sent to your local market.

Such foods usually travel hundreds of miles before coming into your fridge and would have been transferred from freezer to freezer before you get it at home. Also, there could be chances of such foods being given thermal shocks during some part of the transportation process.

All these layers of travel and packaging and freezing is bound to affect the freshness and taste of traditional foods as compared to fresh and mostly unpackaged organic produced grown and sold locally.

Environmentally Safe – As organic foods are not grown using harsh and harmful chemicals, the soil, the water, and the air do not get polluted resulting in a safe environment for one and all. There are true horror stories of how repeated and indiscriminate use of man-made pesticides and fertilizers over a few years has left huge tracts of land completely barren and unsafe for agriculture the soil is totally useless for growing crops. Therefore, organic growing processes are safe from the point of view of being highly environment-friendly.

Animal Welfare – Most non-vegetarians are happy that they are consuming meat and meat products of those animals that have not been subjected to the use of harsh and harmful chemicals. Moreover, there is a sense of contentment that these animals have not been caged or subjected to a miserable way of life. Animal welfare is an important aspect of organic food consumerism, especially in the production of organic meats, organic dairy products, organic fish, and organic poultry.

Organic foods and produce are thus safe for human consumption. In summary, there are studies which prove that they are useful in maintaining and improving human health in the following ways:

- Improves immune system
- Reduces use of pesticides
- Boosts cardiovascular health and protection
- Tastes better than traditionally produced foods
- Improved anti-oxidant capabilities, thereby reducing risk of premature aging, cancer, and other related diseases

- Ensures a safe and healthy environment for the future generation

Chapter Four: Combining Organic Foods and Fasting

Being healthy and fit is the most important thing for all of us. If we are not healthy, we will not be able to perform our daily activities, go to work, support and look after our families, travel, play, and do anything else. How can we start becoming healthy? What is an easy and sensible way to start focusing on our health?

Well, the most important direction you can get to those questions is "What do I eat?" because "we are what we eat!" We have been consuming food from the day we have been born. Our digestive system, our heart, our kidneys, our lungs, and all the organs of our body has been working non-stop from the time we have taken birth on this planet.

How can we give a bit of respite to these organs? One of the best and easiest ways to do this is by fasting. You have already seen the benefits of fasting and the benefits of organic foods. Now, if we can combine the two factors, you are bound to get doubly benefited. Here are some foods you must include in your meals regularly. These foods help you detoxify your body as you fast.

Beverages – Water (purified/filtered), almond milk, coconut kefir, coconut water, vegetable juices

Vegetables – This should be the most important ingredients in your organic meals. Include all kinds of vegetables in cooked and raw form. You can use frozen foods, though truly organic foods don't allow for this. However, make sure you do not include any canned fruits and vegetables as a lot of sugar and salt is added to preserve them in cans.

Fruits – Consume moderately, preferably 1-3 servings a day depending on the kinds of intermittent fasting you decide to go with. You must consume fruits with the following things in mind:

● Cooked or fresh form
● Choose fruits of low glycemic index such as apples, stone fruits, cherries, berries, and all citrus fruits
● You can use dried fruits, but do not eat those that contain sulfites, added sweeteners or oils
● Again, frozen fruit is fine (although it is better to avoid).
● Completely avoid canned fruits

Whole grains – Again consume in moderate amounts and it is best eaten if sprouted. You can include any of the following in your meals:

● Brown rice

- Oats
- Quinoa
- Millets
- Amaranth
- Buckwheat
- Barley

Beans and Legumes – Moderate amounts to be consumed; you can use the dried ones or the fresh ones; canned ones are fine as long as there is no added salt

Nuts and Seeds – Sprouted nuts and seeds are the best forms. However, you can consume dry and the raw form also provided no salt is added.

Vegetables

Here are the vegetables you can choose from for your meals (again choose organic over traditionally grown vegetables and completely avoid canned vegetables with added salt)

Artichokes, Asparagus, Beets, Broccoli, Brussel sprouts, Cabbage, Carrots, Cauliflower, Celery, Collard greens, Corn, Cucumbers, Eggplant, Green beans, Kale, Leeks, Lettuce, Mushrooms, Mustard greens, Okra, Onions, Peppers, Potatoes, Radishes, Rutabagas, Scallions, Spinach, Sprouts, Squash, Sweet potatoes, Tomatoes, Turnips, Yams, Zucchini

Fruits

Here are the fruits you can choose from for your meals (again choose organic over traditionally grown ones and completely avoid canned fruits with added salt/sugar)

Apples, Apricots, Avocados, Bananas, Blackberries, Blueberries, Cantaloupe, Cherries, Coconuts, Cranberries, Dates, Figs, Grapefruit, Grapes, Guava, Honeydew melons, Kiwi, Lemons, Limes, Mangoes, Melons, Nectarines, Oranges, Papayas, Peaches, Pears, Pineapples, Plums, Prunes, Raisins, Raspberries, Strawberries, Tangerines, Watermelon...

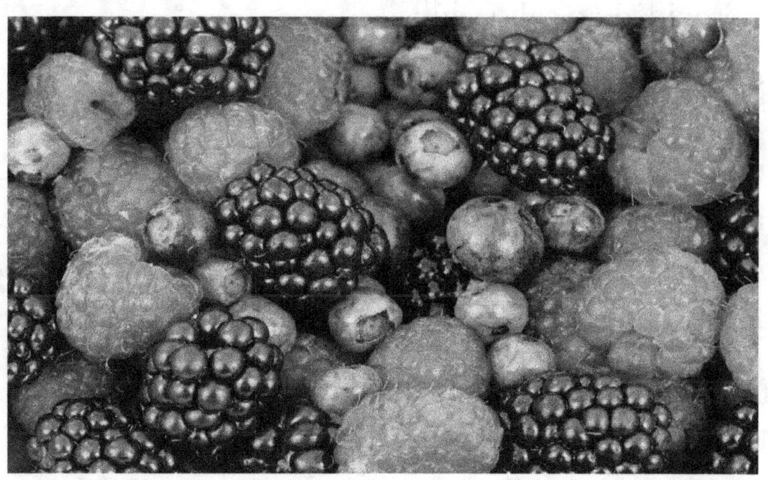

Legumes (preferably organic)

Black beans, Black-eyed peas, Garbanzo beans, Kidney beans, Lentils, Mung beans, Pinto beans, Split peas

Nuts & Seeds (preferably soaked or sprouted unsalted, raw, and organic)

Almonds, Cashews, Chia seeds, Flaxseeds, Pumpkin seeds, Sesame seeds, Sunflower seeds, Walnuts

Whole Grains (preferably organic)

Amaranth, Barley, Brown Rice, Millet, Quinoa, Oats

Liquids

Water (spring, filtered), Vegetable juice (freshly squeezed), Coconut milk, Coconut kefir, Almond milk

Importance of Water in Fasting and Benefits of Water Fasting

Water is an essential commodity of life and nearly 60-70% of our body is composed of water. Water is required for nearly all physiological processes in our system. Water is needed to make new cells, whether skin cells, bone cells, blood cells, etc. Every organ and every organ system in our body needs water to function smoothly and healthily. Water also helps in keeping the lymphatic system functioning well, so that toxins and other wastes are eliminated from the body.

Water is essential for a lot of other functions including:

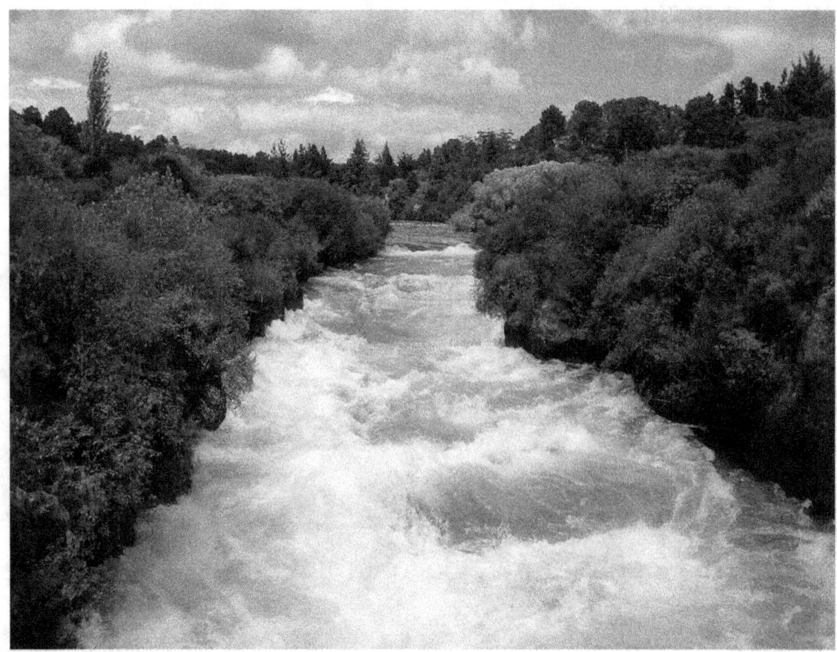

- Lubricating the joints
- Delivering nutrients to the nervous system
- Facilitates the transport of oxygen through blood plasma
- Transports essential nutrients to all cells in your body
- Regulates metabolism
- Helps in digestion
- Regulates body temperature
- Hydrates skin cells and keeps them plump and soft

In fact, there is a fasting methodology that is based only on drinking water for a specified period of time. It is called water fasting and here are some great benefits of water fasting.

Weight loss – Weight loss is something many of us wish for. It is obvious that fasting or not eating will result in reduced body fat. Yet water fasting facilitates weight loss in a unique water. Ketosis is the process wherein your body uses to burn fat cells for its energy needs when no food is supplied. When you drink water during fasting, then this process of ketosis is reached faster than simply from abstaining from eating food. Therefore, stored body fat is used up more quickly with water fasting than fasting without drinking water.

Improved Autophagy – Autophagy is the body's natural process of removing and replacing dysfunctional and unnecessary components, cells, and tissues. Water fasting drives your body into this auto-phagic phase. As fasting reduces calorie intake, the body is compelled to become more selective with regards to which components to repair and which components to eliminate completely, thereby resulting in an effective autophagy.

New Breakthroughs in the Study of Cells in Water

In a study conducted by Dr. Gerald H. Pollack, a professor of Bio-engineering at the University of Washington in Seattle, there was revealing information that challenges our present understanding about how water functions within the cells. We all know that water is needed by our body for hydration. However, this study conducted by Dr. Pollack and his team found that water behaves in a strange way within the cells. Water arranges itself into gel-like layers very close to the cell membrane instead of being in the usual fluid state.

Dr. Pollack refers to this space within the cell as the 'exclusion zone' or EZ. The water in this zone is not the usual H_2O that we know water to be. Here, the gel-like water had the composition of H_3O_2. This zone was referred to as 'exclusion zone' because of its ability to exclude all contaminants and impurities. The water in the EZ is negatively charged and repels contaminants away. While there is a lot more work that needs to be done in this realm, this study holds promise for better understanding detoxification and cell signaling.

Here are some tips on how to do a water fasting:

Consume only good quality water – It is very important that you drink only fresh and good quality water especially during fasting.

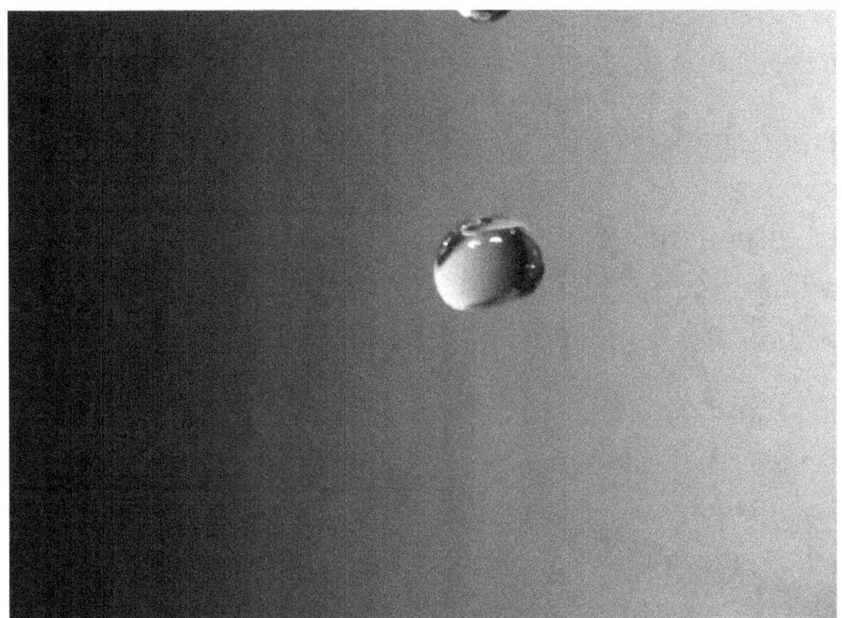

The effects of any toxins and/or contaminants in the water you drink will be magnified in a situation where food is completely absent. Filtered water from a good-quality filter system is good. However, it is even better to use distilled water during fasting.

During distillation, all kinds of harmful organisms and chemicals are thoroughly eliminated.

Arrange your schedule suitably – It would be ideal for you to take time off from work during the water fasting period. It is best to start slowly with a 1-day water fast and with time, gradually increase it to longer durations. It is also advisable to choose a supervised fast under the strict supervision of experts for longer durations to prevent any kind of mishap from happening.

Avoid excessive work and/or physical activities – Fasting is a period of rest. Avoid any kind of activity, including the usual trip to the gym. Of course, it goes without saying not to schedule water fasting regimens when you are preparing for a marathon within the week.

Sleep longer than usual – This is a common side effect of water fasting. Your body will be tired and you will feel like sleeping for a longer time than your usual routine. It is common for people undergoing the water fast to sleep for 12 or more hours in a day.

Expect unpleasant experiences in the first couple of days – The initial 2-3 days will be tough. Unpleasant experiences like gnawing hunger could drive you to increased irritability. You could have headaches and disorienting sensations. You must simply remember that the human body is highly resilient and it will adjust itself to the new routine well. Just be patient with yourself and persist in your efforts.

Indulge in your favorite hobby – Provided it is not physically exerting, indulge in your favorite hobby during water fasting. Reading is a great way to focus on something productive during this time. It is low-energy and focuses your mind without letting it wander without a purpose.

Meditation – Meditating during any fasting regimen reinforces the power of both activities.

So, good organic foods, well-established fasting regimens, and plenty of water can together create magic in your physical, emotional, and spiritual life.

Chapter Five: Intermittent Fasting

We discussed water fasting in the previous chapter, which was a stricter regimen wherein you drank nothing but water during the fasting period, which could last from 1 day to up to a month. This usually requires strict medical supervision for success and to prevent unnecessary mishaps. There is another form of fasting called intermittent fasting that serves the purpose of fasting in the way best described by its name; intermittently.

Intermittent fasting is a deliberating chosen eating pattern wherein there are fixed cycles of eating and fasting. Intermittent fasting does not really focus on the kinds of food you can eat, but instead focuses on when you should eat. Yet, it makes sense to stick to the choices mentioned in the previous chapter during the eating periods of intermittent fasting regimens.

There are different methods and types of intermittent fasting. All these types divide the day or the week into periods of eating or periods of fasting. It is true that nearly everyone fasts for a few hours every 24 hours; when they sleep. Intermittent fasting simply requires you to extend this natural fasting period to last a little more.

An example would be to skip breakfast and eat lunch (your first meal of the day) at 12 noon and dinner at 8

PM. This means you will be fasting for 16 hours (fasting period) and you will have a window of 8 hours (the eating period) during which time you will have two meals. The calorie intake of the breakfast is completely eliminated, resulting in a lesser calorie intake than if you were not fasting. Of course, this works only when the calorie intake for lunch and dinner stays at the usual amount and does not make up for the lost calories of the skipped breakfast. This is a popular method of intermittent fasting and is called the 16/8 method.

Similarly, there are other types of intermittent fasting. During the fasting periods, it is important to keep out calorie intake completely, although non-alcoholic beverages like tea, coffee, water, etc. are allowed. It goes without saying that there should not be any added sugar content in the beverages.

Intermittent fasting is a popular form of an eating pattern wherein you have strictly laid-down eating and fasting periods. Before we go into the types of intermittent fasting, let us look at some of the benefits of this method of fasting.

Benefits of Intermittent Fasting

Increased fat loss – Intermittent fasting helps you to get lean as your body will draw its energy from stored fat during the fasting periods. Stubborn fat will be shifted once you have an achieved a low body-fat percentage. Even for people with a significantly higher body-fat percentage, weight loss is one of the major benefits of intermittent fasting. You will see these results if you stay committed to the regimen even for a short period of time.

Less cravings – While fat loss is a fabulous benefit by itself, intermittent fasting will also reduce unnecessary cravings driven by the usual fasting methods. Intermittent fasting teaches you to discern between real hunger and a simple whim to eat something. It suppresses hunger and as you follow the chosen regimen diligently, you will find yourself feeling satiated after eating the first meal after the fast without indulging in overeating.

Improved insulin sensitivity – When you fast for 16 hours and you partake of your first meal, your body will become more sensitive to insulin, resulting in stable levels of this critical hormone which otherwise can play havoc in your life. Insulin levels are likely to fluctuate less which, in turn, also improves protein synthesis as this is also controlled by insulin. Improved insulin sensitivity will result in lesser cravings and a heightened appreciation for the food you have eaten.

Better cognitive state – It is a myth that fasting will result in sluggishness and fatigue. After a fasted state, you will feel more alert and capable of performing better because your brain is in a state of heightened alertness because of the lack of food. Blood is not being pumped to the digestive system because there is no food to be digested. This blood is instead channeled to the other parts of the body, such as muscles (if you are doing a physical workout) or your brain (if you are involved in some mind activity) which will make you feel more alert and active than when your stomach is full of food.

Now, let us look at some of the most popular types of intermittent fasting and their features.

The 16/8 Method

This method has been discussed in brief as an example above. Let us look at it in a bit more detail. This method was popularized by Martin Berkhan, the fitness expert.

This type involves fasting periods that last 14-16 hours and eating periods that last 8-10 hours. During the eating period, you can have 2, 3, or more meals fit in. The easiest form of this type is to eat nothing after dinner and skip breakfast the next morning; your lunch at noon will be your first meal of the day.

So, for example, if you finish dinner at 8 PM, then don't eat anything until lunch the next day at 12 noon. This will effectively result in 16 hours of fasting, which is sufficient time for ketosis to set in and some amount of body fats to be burned for calorie needs.

This might appear to be a difficult thing to do for people who love their breakfast. However, many people who skip breakfast actually eat this way. Drinking water, coffee, and tea during fasting periods can help in managing hunger pangs although once your body gets used to this routine, the hunger pangs will also disappear.

Another important thing to keep in mind is to stick to healthy meals during the eating periods and make a conscious effort not make up for the loss of calories resulting from the skipped meal. Stick to a low-carb diet and ensure you get in plenty of vegetables, both raw and cooked. Avoid excessive sugar in your tea and coffee, which you are allowed even during the fasting periods. By the way, feel free to chew sugar-free gum during the fasting period.

The 5/2 Method

This method involves eating normally on five days of the week and keeping calorie intake at 500-600 on 2 days of the week. This method is referred to as the Fast Diet and was popularized by Dr. Michael Mosley, a doctor and a British journalist. On the two fasting days, women are recommended to restrict their meals to 2 meals of 250 calories each resulting in 500 calories for the day. Men are recommended to restrict their calorie intake to 600 through two meals of 300 calories each.

In this method, you will never have to go through any day without food. The fast days are merely restricted to the amount of calorie intake. So, even on fast days, you are allowed to eat small meals totaling to not more than 500-600 calories, which is about a quarter of our daily calorie requirements.

You can eat anything you like on fast days provided you stick to the restricted calories recommended for those days. However, soups, salads, and plenty of water are the recommended meals for fasting days

The fast days can be any two days of the week. So, it is fine to choose a Monday and a Thursday or a Tuesday and a Friday or anything else you like. Keeping two consecutive days could be more difficult to adhere to as restricting calorie intake consecutively can be quite challenging. Taking breaks in between the two days can be a good thing to ensure commitment.

Like all fasting methods, avoiding rigorous physical activity is a good idea here too.

Eat-Stop-Eat

This method involves a 24-hour fast for 1-2 days a week. Brad Pilon, the fitness expert, is given the credit for popularizing this method. Fasting after the dinner on one day until the dinner on the next day is a 24-hour regimen. For example, if you have eaten dinner on Monday at 8

PM, you will not eat anything until dinner at 8 PM on Tuesday. You can do this from breakfast to breakfast or lunch to lunch; whatever suits you. Again, water, tea, coffee (with very little or no sugar) is allowed during the fasting periods but absolutely no solid food.

Here too, when you eat after the 24-hour fast, it is important to eat only what you have promised yourself. Do not make up for the lost calories. This is especially important for people following this regimen to lose weight. Here are some tips for this method of intermittent fasting:

Don't Panic about Loss of Water and Muscle – There are a lot of myths floating around about this method of fasting including that one tends to lose muscle and water instead of fat. Do not believe these myths. You will only lose fat and you will definitely not lose muscle. Ensure you drink plenty of water to stay hydrated.

Begin the Fast after Dinner – Suppose you finish dinner at around 7 PM and you work until about 9 PM and go to sleep sufficiently satiated. When you wake up the next morning at 7 AM, you have already completed half the 24 hours. This can be highly motivated in addition to the enticement of being able to eat before you go to sleep for the night again. Moreover, since you have finished an early dinner at 7 PM, you will sleep better.

Drink Lots of Water – Filling your stomach with water, tea, and coffee without sugar can make you overcome hunger pangs easily, especially when you know you will eat before you go to sleep.

Eat Normal Sized Meals after the Fast – Eat the same amount of food that you would eat if you had not been fasting. Your meal after the fast should not be more than the usual. Again, do not eat junk foods, processed foods, etc. Eat normal-sized wholesome meals with plenty of vegetables and low-carb cereals.

Do Not Break Your Fast for Hunger – Intermittent fasting helps us discipline our body and mind. Find ways and means to manage your hunger pangs. Do not give in to temptation and do not break your commitment to fast because you are feeling hungry.

Ensure the 24-Hour Regimen Is Not For More Than 2 Days a Week – Using this method for more than 2 days a week is not a good idea. A 2-day fast cuts calorie intake by 30%. More than 30% can result in lowered strength and energy leaving you drained and unhappy, which, in turn, can result in overeating.

Commit For At Least 2 Months – If you wish to see any kind of obvious results like a significant amount of weight loss, you must commit yourself to at least 2 months of this regimen. It takes your body 2 months to get used to this regimen and actually show you the desired outcomes.

Chapter Six: Intermittent Fasting – Continued

Alternate-Day Fasting

As the name suggests, this type requires fasting to be done every other day. There are different versions of this type. While some use water fasting, others restrict calorie intake to 500 on the fasting days. Many of the research studies conducted on intermittent fasting used this format to arrive at both the positive and negative conclusions.

A complete fast every other day may not be a wise thing for beginners as it can be quite extreme. This method entails you to go to bed with hunger pangs gnawing for many days in the week and it can be a very unpleasant experience. Undergoing this experience often can lead to a breakdown in commitment levels leading to failure of the fasting regimen.

You could look at this method, perhaps, after achieving some kind of mastery in one of the easier methods discussed earlier. Here are some advantages and disadvantage of the alternate-day fasting method:

Advantages

- It helps you lose weight effectively and quickly as your body is deprived of calorie intake so often that it is pushed to use up accumulated fat for its energy requirements.

- Studies have proved that this method is excellent to prevent the onset of chronic diseases such as diabetes, cancers, and cardiovascular problems

- This method can actually be easy to follow, especially in the short-term. Not having to worry about food every other day can be a liberating experience which could work for some time.

Disadvantages

- Committing to this method of intermittent fasting can be a challenging thing in the long-term horizon

- The lack of nutrition could push you to avoid all kinds of physical activities which could deter your journey to a fit life

The Warrior Diet

Ori Hofmekler, a famous fitness expert popularized the Warrior Diet. This kind of intermittent fasting involves consuming very little amounts of raw vegetables and fruits throughout the day and eating one big meal at night. That is to say, you fast the entire day and feast during dinner time. The Warrior Diet also recommends you to adhere to the Paleo Diet (as followed by our cavemen ancestors) and eat unprocessed foods as possibly close to what is available in nature.

The following guidelines for the 'feasting' dinner will help in the success of the Warrior Diet:

- Avoid all kinds of processed foods

- Eat only organic and natural foods including whole grains, grass-fed meats, etc.

- All frozen and 'packaged' foods are to be avoided as well.

- Plastic packaged foods should not be consumed since plastic fibers are known to contain chemicals that behave like estrogen in the body

- Avoid alcohol as much as possible as it frees up your liver to focus on productive work that helps in keeping your body fit and healthy

- Keep carbs for the last meal as this will help in stabilizing blood sugar levels and also help you go through the next day without many carbs until dinner time

- Varying between high-protein and high-fat diets alternately helps you optimize the effect of this diet

Skipping Meals at Your Convenience

This is, perhaps, the easiest form of intermittent fasting as it requires almost no planning from your end. This method entails you to skip meals as and when you feel like it, especially when you are not hungry. There are experts who believe that 'eating every four hours' to avoid starvation is a myth that some scientists and nutritionists have built up.

The human body is very well equipped to handle long periods of starvation such as those experienced during famines and catastrophes. So, it is perfectly alright to miss your breakfast and eat a healthy lunch. Just keep in mind not to overeat your lunch because you have skipped your breakfast. It's all in the mind. Your body will do as your mind wills it to. Here are some good reasons for skipping breakfast:

Breakfast Does Not Affect Your Metabolism – There are experts who claim that eating small meals at frequent intervals can increase metabolism. However, there are studies which reveal that such kind of eating does not increase metabolism. In fact, Brad Pilon and Martin Berkhan, proponents of intermittent fasting have been able to prove that fasting increases metabolism and not frequent and small meals.

Breakfast Does Not Stop Breakdown of Muscle – Starvation mode resulting in muscle loss is a myth. You will not lose out muscle if you don't eat every 3-4 hours because your muscles do not need proteins so frequently. It is more important to get protein before the workout mode rather than ensure you get protein every 3 hours through frequent meals.

Breakfast Does Not Manage Blood Sugar Levels Well – The reason given for eating breakfast is to raise your blood-sugar levels after the night's fast so that insulin levels are stabilized. But this is not really what is happening in the body. Insulin is responsible for muscle growth and fat storage. Fasting decreases the insulin levels in your blood, thereby increasing your body's sensitivity far more significantly than eating every 3 hours.

Breakfast Increases Hunger – There are many people who get hungrier than usual if they eat breakfast. This could be an advantage or disadvantage depending on whether you want to gain weight or lose fat:

Increased hunger because of eating breakfast is great for weight gain as skinny guys who want to put on weight will be able to meet their calorific requirements for the day.

Increased hunger because of eating breakfast is not good at all if you are looking at fat loss as there is no increased metabolism because of eating breakfast and you will have to restrict food choices throughout the day which can be very challenging most of the time

Breakfast is Actually Unnatural – Look at the healthiest of our ancestors, the cavemen. They couldn't have eaten a hearty breakfast as soon as they got up in the morning. They probably would have had to hunt before they even got food to eat!

Therefore, breakfast does not directly improve your health. However, if used sensibly, it can create healthy eating habits. So, choose the intermittent fasting that suits you best and start following it. Listen to your body and you will be fine!

Bonus Chapter: The most simple and best diet on Earth

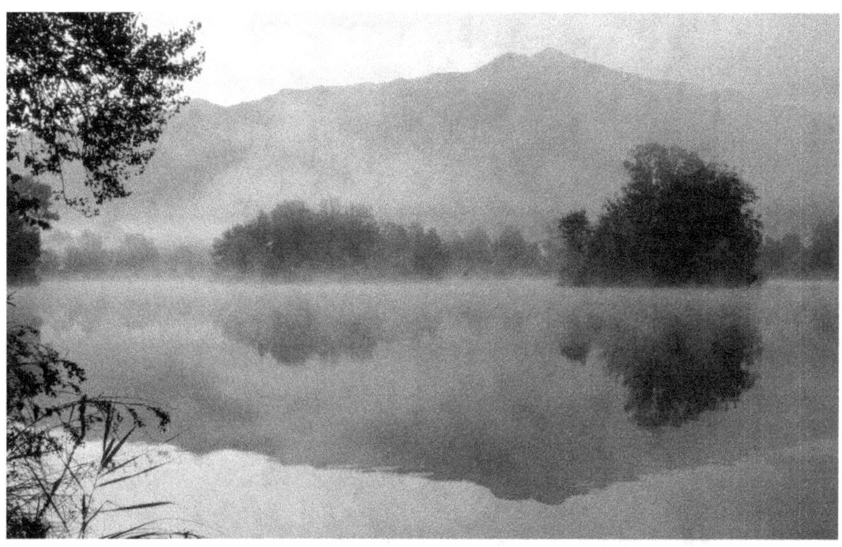

As we have seen different fasting methods, and because there are as many ways as individuals on this planet, I would like to share with you some of my own personal ways. Each of us has his preference when it comes to eating, but it's also food habits. Sometimes we just eat the same things over and over because we know we like it and we know how to cook it, and forget to try a new thing.

By sharing my knowledge on this diet, I really want to light up your food life experience.

This diet is my base nourishment. I keep this main source of ingredients, and adding various kind of herbs and spices.

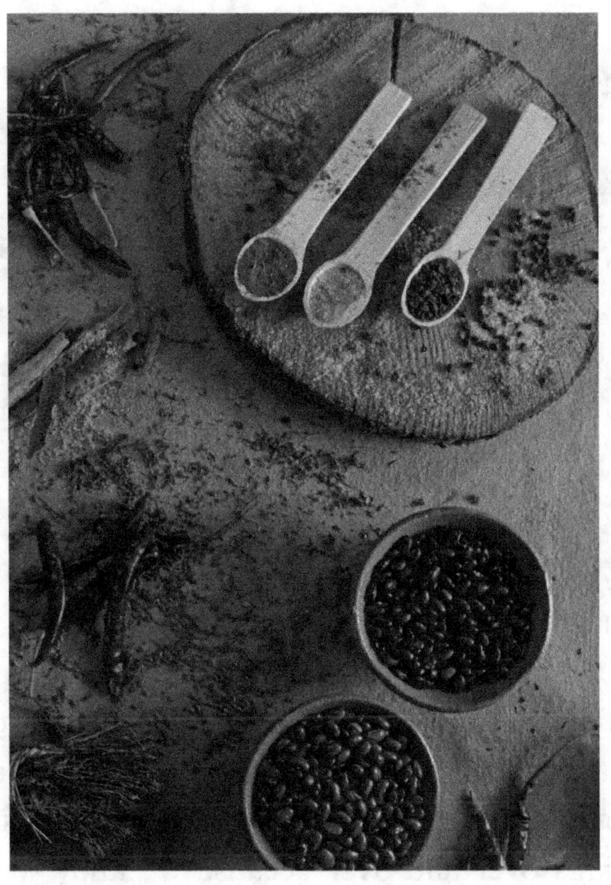

Basic ingredients of the Diet:

- Potatoes (Sweet, Red, Yellow)

- Rice (Try different kind)

- Beans (Black, Red, Peas...)

- Lentils

- Avocados

- Tomatoes

- Onions, Garlic, Shallots

- Bananas

- Fruits (All kind)

- Coconut Oil, Olive Oil

- Himalayan Pink Salt

- Spices (All kind)

- Mint, Basil

Make sure everything come from the Earth, Organic ingredients.

With this Diet, you will feel satisfied; this is fulfilling, nourishing and last but not least very tasty ! You can prepare your everyday meals with this simple base. And adjust with your flavors preference.

How to prepare your meal

Cook the potatoes:

Rinse the potatoes. Don't remove the skin, it contains a lot of good nutrients for your body.

Boil the potatoes in water (better with pure water, from moving source if possible)

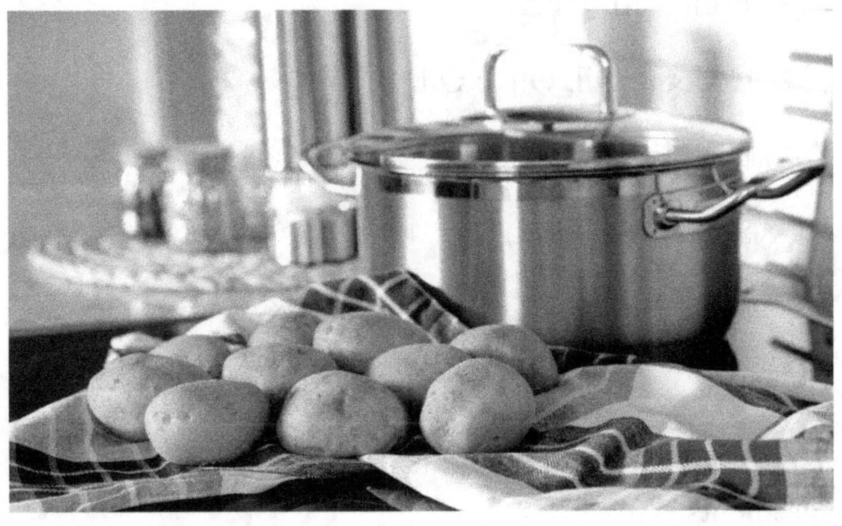

The potato is a great source of nutrients, and it's very fulfilling. That's why I recommend it in this base diet.

But you can alternate with:

- Rice (Brown, White, Black, Red...)

- Lentils (tasty with mushrooms and onions)

- Black beans (tasty with corn and onions)

Add Coconut Oil or Olive Oil to sweet your meal.

Prepare the guacamole:

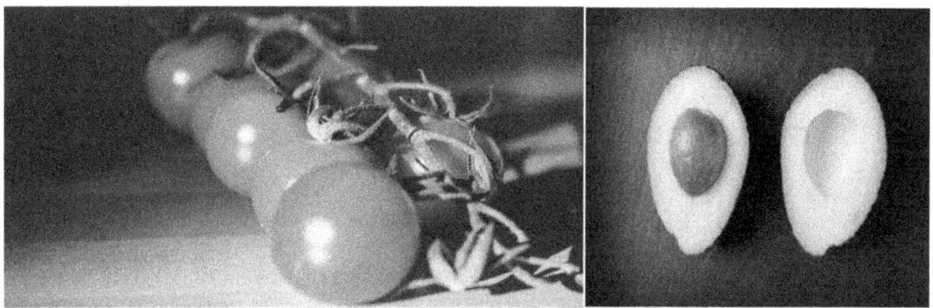

Cut avocados and tomatoes in small dices.

In a bowl, Mix the avocados with tomatoes (basic guacamole)

You can add small dices of onions, shallots or garlic if you like. Add pink Himalayan salt.

Then you can join different kind of spices or herbs of your choice.

Personally I love put turmeric or cayenne pepper powder inside, even with mint or basil it's delicious. But you can try with all bunch of different things, with every ingredient that you like or that come in your mind.

Feel free to mix different kind of spices and herbs and try all you can imagine. It's a very good creativity exercise in the same time, and your tongue will thank you for experimenting new flavors. Plus you can change every day, and try a new taste at every meal!

Once your ingredients choice is done:

Stir the mix as much as you like.

More you will stir it, more the juice of the tomatoes will incorporate the avocado. And more it will become like a sauce.

Once the potatoes are boiled, open it in two or cut it in dices, serve it on a plate or bowl, and put the guacamole over or at side. Adjust your taste with salt.

You can take a moment to thank the Earth, then eat and enjoy your meal!

After your meal, you can drink hot herbal tea if you like. It is great for digestion. You can also drink water with lemon juice.

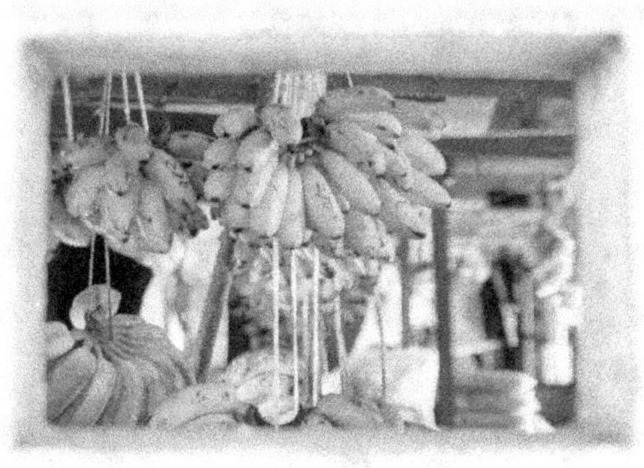

And if your still a bit hungry, you can complete it with bananas. Raw bananas or mixed with coconut (milk, oil, shreds, powder), you can even add dark chocolate or cocoa.

Then besides your meals, feel free to eat different kind of nuts. Moreover, eat fruits all day long! Make sure they are organic. Do not overeat, and try to identify and recognize what your body need at that time. So you can fulfilling yourself with the right ingredient.

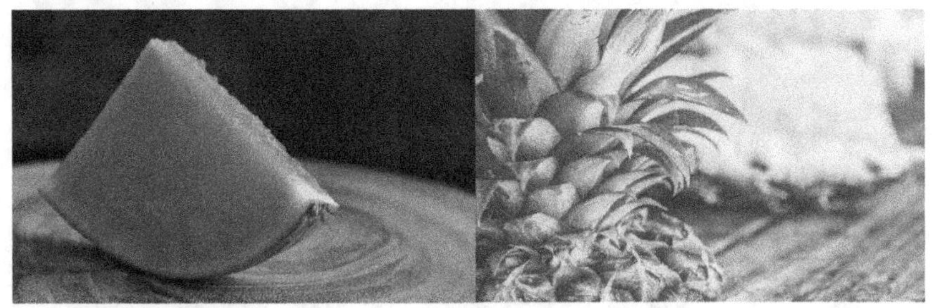

Easy to digest:

One of the great advantage of this diet, is its digestion. Depending of your appetite, you can eat a lot in fulfilling quantities and still digest fluently. After your meal, energy will circulate in your body. You are not going to feel low after eating, the digestion will flow with ease that you almost will not noticed it. And you will remember how you sprawled on the couch just after swallowed a big junk food fat meal. All the energy not used for the digestion will be available for multiple activities, you will also notice the clarity of your mind, for mental work for example.

Besides, your are not going to be thirsty, or little, essentially because of the juice of tomatoes. Comparing with heavy food like cheese or meat that dehydrates your body, it will conversely hydrates your body immediately. If you're nevertheless thirsty, you can drink hot herbal tea or eat aqueous fruits (like watermelons, peaches, grapes, strawberries, pineapples, kiwis,...)

Likewise, it is easier to relieve oneself. For those with transit problems, it is a good way to fluidize the intestinal transit. Your body will process the meal naturally with ease, it will take less effort to digest.

If you are close to Nature, you can go outside, and thank the nature back with your poop. So we can respect the circle of life.

Developing Melanin:

To rejuvenate the body, the DNA must regenerate. To regenerate, the DNA need sun light. Organic Sun light. With this diet, you are helping your melanin to develop itself. Your epidermis will be prepared and your skin will be apt to receive the sun beams. The Melanin repair the DNA, actually Melanin is the Universe itself, at its purest form. Our body is a holographic Universe. So by developing our melanin, we heal and purify our DNA.

You going to tan easily, yes actually more you eat naturally with organic ingredients that come from the earth, more you are going to receive the sun with ease. Prepare your body to welcome the sun beams, forget sunburns experience!

More you take sunlight, more you will produce melanin. And more you will develop your melanin, more you can go under the sun and receive sun light fluently. But with chemicals inside you (through toxic food), your melanin can not develop properly. That's why have a healthy and clean diet is primordial. If your blood and melanin is not clean and pure, you will probably get sunburns (it depend of your skin, it's relative for each individual). A sunburn is not a punishment from the sun, it is more like a warning or a lesson to make you realize your body is not enough clean inside, so you have to change something.

It goes deeper actually, melanin allows us to connect to what we really are, the universe itself. More your melanin will be developed, more you will be able to communicate with the sun, and so with the Universe. Yes it is a communication, the sun is sending you light and you are receiving it.

Being in tune with the Universe is being in tune with yourself, that means in clean health, in good shape mentally, physically and spiritually.

Bonus Tip: How to remove bad odor from your Body

To end up this book, I would like to share with you some tips, it look likes a bit off topic, but it is really all connected when it comes to the body.

Most people on this planet have had a sweaty and stinking body experience, sometimes or often. I hope I will help you dealing with that for your own body.

Actually, our body produce a natural odor, a unique one. But we almost forgot it nowadays, we cover ourselves with lotions, fragrances, sunscreen and all kind of chemicals things. With these unnatural habits, it's like we want to hide our proper and real odor.

If you eat some toxic or unnatural food, your body will process it by rejecting it. Remember that the body is very intelligent and will always do the right thing to sustain itself. In this case it just want to get rid of this unnecessary excess.

So the main exit door that the body will use to remove this surplus is the armpits. That's why we usually sweat and smell bad the most in this area.

The following process is an external technique to avoid smelling bad from armpits. But remember that the ultimate way to not smelling bad is internal, don't put bad things in your body and you will not smell bad. Simple as that.

My simple tip:

First wash your armpits with water (avoid shower gel or chemical lotions) then dry it. Make sure you're not irritated or cut on this area.

Then take an organic lemon, cut it and press it to get some juice in your hand. Apply the juice all over your armpits. Then let it breathe a moment, without clothes on.

Done.

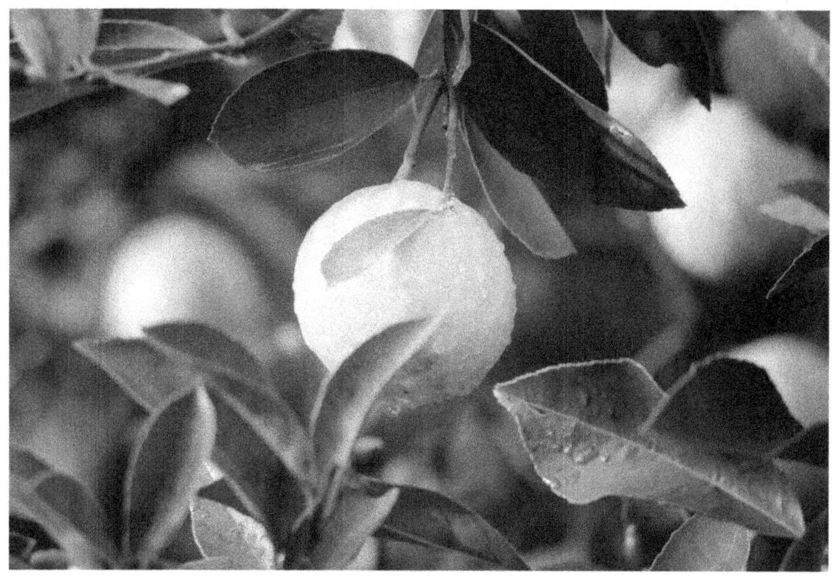

The action of lemon is very powerful, it will neutralize bad odor that come from your body.

Do it as much as you need, one application will be effective for 3 or 4 days usually. But that depend of what kind of food you eat, healthier it will be, smoother the odor will be.

With this technique, your odor will be kind of neutral, and gradually you will get your real odor back. And don't worry you will not smell lemon all day! Just at the application time.

According to what you eat and by using this tip, you are going to notice the change of your odor.

Conclusion

All diseases that we notice in our society are consequences of our way of life, and food is one of these factors, a major one.

Now that you know about the benefits and the various methods of fasting including intermittent fasting and the appropriate food to integrate. I would like to finish this book with a few words of caution. Like all things in the world, there needs to be a balance in the way you handle your intermittent fasting process. It requires thought, commitment and self-awareness.

When you use simpler and easier-to-follow intermittent fasting methods, remember the following tips:

- Listen to your body; if it is telling you it cannot take it, then stop your regimen.
- Take things gradually. Start with something very simple, See how it goes and slowly increase your intensity of fasting. Never hesitate to get back to normal if it doesn't suit you.
- The healthy in fasting lies in 'healthy fasting.' Avoid going overboard and be sensible and reasonable with your expectations.

Here are some precautionary measures you should take to ensure nothing untoward happens:

While it is ideal for everyone to consult their physician before embarking on any fasting journey, the following people should necessarily consult their doctor(s) before undertaking any fasting regimen:

- People who are extremely frail
- People with a compromised or weakened immunity
- People with eating problems and disorders
- People who are dependent on medication for diabetes, hypertension, or other problems
- People who are on medication for all chronic ailments including but not limited to heart diseases, etc.

While it is possible to undertake fasting regimens for most disorders, the more serious the ailment, the more medical supervision is needed. People on prescription medicines could have varying dietary needs every day and it is important to ensure your food intake matches these dietary requirements failing which you could land in trouble.

For example, if you are on medications to lower hypertension, then fasting itself could help with this. Consequently, it is possible that your doctor lowers your dosage to make up for it. If you didn't consult your doctor, the double effects of fasting and the medication could lower your blood pressure below recommended levels which could prove harmful!

For longer-term and rarer forms of water fasting, it is imperative that you use the services of an established and well-reputed fasting clinic because complications which cannot be managed at home could arise. For example, continued water fasting might lower electrolyte levels in your body which requires immediate medical attention. Long-term fasting regimens are best done at approved clinics under strict medical supervision.

While these precautions are mandatory, you must also remember the multiple benefits listed in this book about fasting. So, go ahead, start small, persist in your efforts, and reap the benefits of your commitment sooner than later.

To conclude, in your fasting process, the most important thing to do is study yourself. More you are going to progress in your journey and more you will start to notice what you can afford in term of fasting time, quantities, and kind of food. And also what you can afford, You have to respect the steps, if your body is not ready to experiment something you must know it. You are going to learn how your body respond at each step you do.

Of course medicine will give you some precautions and advises, but only you will know if you can do it. Be responsible of your own actions. Be your own doctor.

Remember, in our way of life, food is a major factor for healing and creating a good balance of energy, but it's not the only one. Many other elements come into play, but we will see that an other time.

Resources

http://www.telegraph.co.uk/lifestyle/11524808/The-history-of-fasting.html

http://www.allaboutfasting.com/benefits-of-fasting.html

https://www.globalhealingcenter.com/natural-health/health-benefits-of-fasting/

https://www.organicfacts.net/health-benefits/other/health-benefits-of-fasting.html

http://www.rawfoodexplained.com/when-to-employ-fasting/does-fasting-cure-disease.html

https://breakingmuscle.com/healthy-eating/intermittent-fasting-for-athletes-the-why-and-how

https://www.healthline.com/nutrition/intermittent-fasting-and-weight-loss#section1

http://www.thehealersjournal.com/2013/04/15/fasting-effects-healing-the-brain-nervous-endocrine-system/

https://www.organicfacts.net/organic-products/organic-food/health-benefits-of-organic-food.html

http://runawayleg.com/organic-fasting/

http://www.organicauthority.com/health/skip-the-juice-diet-10-natural-food-detox.html, https://draxe.com/daniel-fast/

https://www.globalhealingcenter.com/natural-health/health-benefits-of-water-fasting/

https://www.healthline.com/nutrition/10-health-benefits-of-intermittent-fasting#section6

https://draxe.com/benefits-fasting/

https://www.myprotein.com/thezone/nutrition/intermittent-fasting-lean-gains-168/

https://www.healthline.com/nutrition/6-ways-to-do-intermittent-fasting#section1

https://the5-2dietbook.com/basics

https://stronglifts.com/eat-stop-eat-7-tips-to-make-intermittent-fasting-easier/

https://draxe.com/alternate-day-fasting/

https://www.lifejacks.com/warrior-diet-well-founded-intermittent-fasting-plan/

https://www.healthline.com/nutrition/6-ways-to-do-intermittent-fasting#section3

https://stronglifts.com/7-reasons-why-you-should-not-eat-breakfast/

http://www.allaboutfasting.com/healthy-fasting.html

9 781721 083831